Cover design by: Samantha Munguia

This book is dedicated to my family and friends. I could not have done it without your support.

Thank you

CONTENTS

WHAT IS THIS BOOK ABOUT?

I am going to share with you what I have learned on my weight loss journey while trying to be as concise as possible. In this book, I cover what I believe are the most important things I have learned from years of trial and error. There will also be a story or two in here, which I hope will help you remember some of the more important details. But first, I will share a little about myself so you know I'm not a random person writing about weight loss.

ABOUT THE AUTHOR

First off, I never imagined I would be writing an "About the Author" section, let alone a book. Then again, I never imagined I would have lost 90 pounds or that I would ever run a full marathon. It just goes to prove that really nothing is impossible.

I have struggled with weight loss for most of my life. I tried a variety of DIEts over the years. Most with little to no success. The ones that worked were hard to maintain and would always bring temporary results. I would ultimately go back to old habits and often put on more weight than what I managed to lose.

In 2014, I weighed around 269 pounds, a few pounds away from morbidly obese. It was time for a change. I grew tired of not being comfortable with myself and did not want to deal with health issues accompanied by obesity for the rest of my life. I ended up going to a nutritionist who finally helped me understand how to lose weight. I dropped close to 90 pounds in five years. However, it was not five years of constant weight loss. After I lost the first 50 or so pounds, I became a little complacent. I maintained that weight for a while until I finally got back on track. In 2019, I weighed 178 pounds and was in the best shape of my life. I completed the Spartan Trifecta and ran a full marathon. Getting in shape and losing weight was not easy.

I am still trying to better myself daily. Even though I want to lose a couple more pounds, I've gathered enough knowledge and experience to help others out there who are struggling as I did. I hope there is something in this book that can help you.

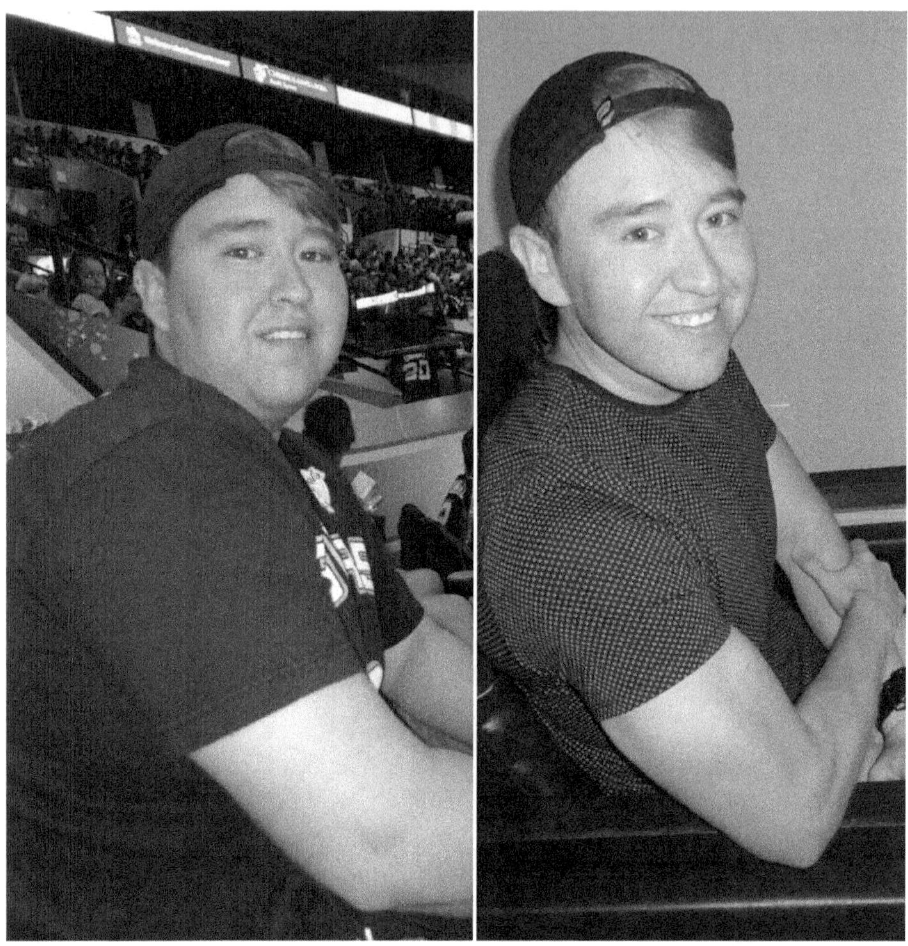

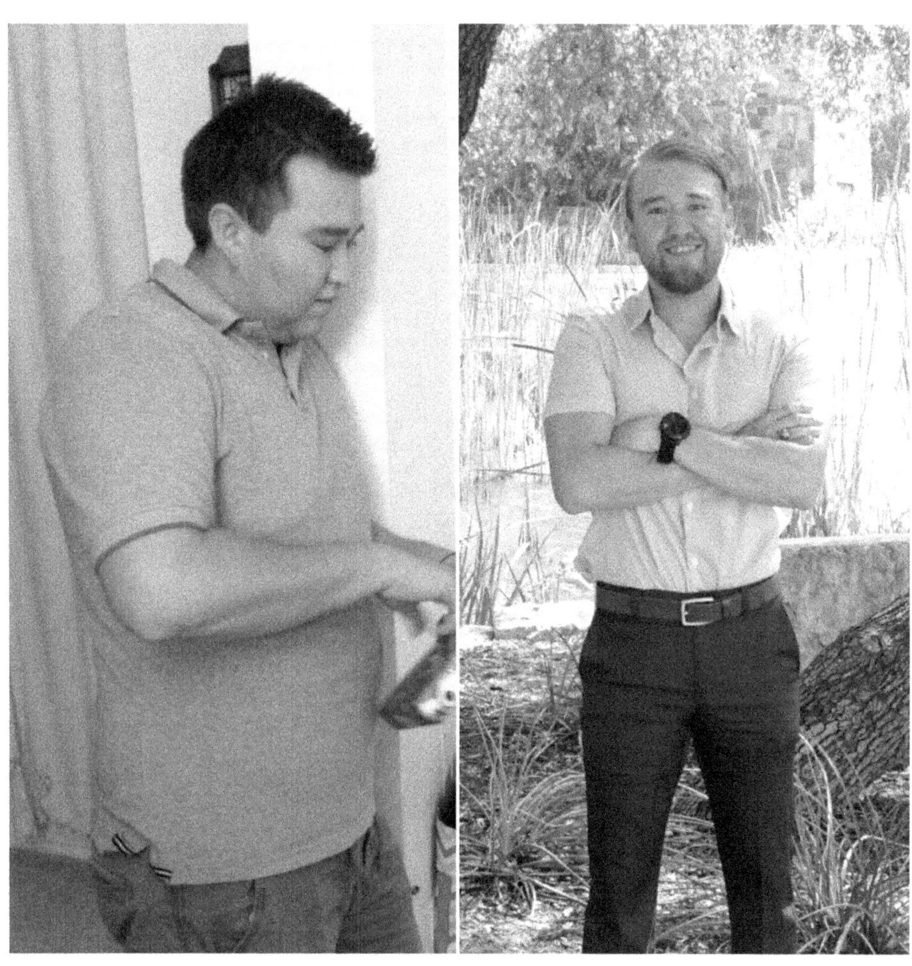

I strongly believe that if I can do it, anyone can do it. Yes, that includes **YOU**!

Let's get started.

TRUTH HURTS

Weight loss is hard.

There is no magic pill. There is no easy, fast solution. Sorry. You are going to have to struggle with it, and it is going to take some time. However, it is not impossible and in the end, it will all be worth it. Trust me.

HI, HELLO, WHAT?

You don't need to exercise to lose weight.

Yes, you read that right. Exercise plays an important factor in weight loss, but you can lose weight simply by controlling your DIEt.

Your body will burn around 2,000 calories, a rough estimate, simply by waking up and binge-watching your favorite show. You might be physically doing nothing, but your body consumes that energy to keep you alive. Cool, science.

So basically, if your weight loss journey consisted only of waking up and doing nothing all day while eating less than 2,000 calories, you would successfully lose weight. To get a closer estimate of the number of calories your body uses to simply keep you alive, you need to consider other variables. I will elaborate in another chapter.

Approximately, the first 20 pounds I lost were mainly attributed to changes in my DIEt. The extent of my exercise came from walking around campus at UTSA. It wasn't anything too strenuous.

DIEt is the is the important factor in weight loss!!

DIEt is the is the important factor in weight loss!!

MAGIC OF SCIENCE

Weight loss is not magic; it's simply science. To lose weight, you just need to be in a caloric deficit. In other words, you need to eat fewer calories than what your body needs so that it's forced to burn off excess fat for energy.

Never truly understanding the science behind weight loss always hindered my success. Maybe that's a little weird, but I have a bachelor's degree in Mechanical Engineering. I'm wired to figure out how things work. I am going to explain some key terms and concepts that I wish I knew a long time ago to help you understand the science of weight loss.

However, if you are not interested in the math behind figuring out your calorie goal or macronutrients, then feel free to skip the next two chapters. If you skip ahead, just assume it's magic and go with the flow. You won't have to compute anything later, so you don't need this information. However, I strongly believe it's helpful to know what is going on inside your body.

CALORIES

The idea of eating fewer than 2,000 calories a day to lose weight didn't appear out of thin air. If you've ever glanced at a nutrition label, you probably read the disclaimer that says, "2,000 calories a day is used for general nutrition advice." That number was chosen by the Food and Drug Administration (FDA) to give you an idea of how many calories to base your diet on.

The number of calories your body needs to stay alive while at rest is called the Basal Metabolic Rate (BMR). Your BMR depends on variables such as gender, age, height, and weight. There have been several equations developed over the years to approximate your BMR.

The most common formula used to find your BMR is the Harris-Benedict Equation; it is what I used to calculate my BMR which will be shown down below. You can research other equations or even use an online calculator to calculate your BMR and see how much the values differ. It's kind of fun! Well, it was fun for me. One of my engineering professors used to tell us, "I can do something with some data, but I can do nothing with no data." Any method you chose to find your BMR is going to be an estimate, but you will at least have a number to start with.

Use the Harris-Benedict Equation below to calculate your own. Note there is a different equation for men and women. BMR value will usually be much higher for men.

Men: *BMR = 66 + (6.23 x weight in pounds) + (12.7 x height in inches) – (6.8 x age in years)*

Women: *BMR = 655 + (4.35 x weight in pounds) + (4.7 x height in inches) – (4.7 x age in years)*

Cool, we found our BMR! Your BMR will change as your weight changes and will be different from mine. Again, it will depend on gender, age, weight, and height.

My current BMR is 1,932 calories, which means if I consume 1,932 calories daily over time, I will **MAINTAIN** my current weight. If I consume less than 1,932 calories daily over time, I will **LOSE** weight. If I consume over 1,932 calories daily over time, I will **GAIN** weight. However, all these cases are under the assumption that I'm not partaking in any physical activity.

Weight loss = Caloric Deficit

That's good to know, but how much of a caloric deficit must we maintain to lose weight?

According to the Mayo Clinic, to realistically lose weight and keep it off long term, it's recommended you aim to lose one to two pounds per week. It is not healthy to lose weight too quickly.

When I first started my weight loss journey, I could easily drop more than the recommended two pounds a week. Don't worry if you drop more than two pounds per week for a while; it probably has to do with the aggressive change in your DIEt. After a while, everything slows down. If I managed to lose two pounds per week right now, I would be overjoyed with happiness. As you get in better shape it's more difficult to lose weight. You will reach several plateaus and will need to be more strict with your DIEt and exercise to overcome them.

In 1958, Max Wishnofsky concluded it takes 3,500 calories to burn one pound of fat. More recent studies show the number might be a little flawed because he did not account for other important factors. However, it's still a good estimate to use.

According to that caloric estimate, we can conclude you need to be at a 500-calorie deficit per day to lose one pound of fat in a week. One pound of fat per week doesn't sound all that great, but there are 52 weeks in a year. That equates to 52 pounds lost in one year. If you are aiming to lose two pounds per week, we are looking at 104 pounds lost in one year! Of course, losing 52 pounds in a year would be in a perfect world. Everyone will get different results, but theoretically, those are the tangible results.

Alright, cool. We are going to aim to lose one to two pounds of fat per week. With my current BMR at 1,932 calories, I would have to eat 1,432 calories per day to lose one pound of fat in a week.

$$1,932 - 500 = 1,432 \ cal/day$$

If I want to lose two pounds per week, I would have to eat 932 calories daily.

$$1,932-1,000=932 \; cal/day$$

I don't know about you, but it would be torture for me if I had to only consume 932 calories in one day to lose two pounds of fat per week. I might be able to eat 1,432 calories per day, but I would be miserable. Luckily, this caloric estimate is based on my BMR only. This estimate assumes that I am just going to sit on my couch all day.

The number we want to know is our Total Daily Energy Expenditure (TDEE). We can find this value by multiplying our BMR value by an activity multiplier. Just like the BMR, there are several methods to find your activity multiplier. Go online and search "TDEE calculator." If you do, calculating your BMR was not necessary. However, understanding where all these numbers are coming from is what helped me truly understand weight loss.

Okay, time for some more math. I am using multiplier values published in an article by Kansas State University titled "Physical Activity and Controlling Weight." The results can be seen in the table below. Again, the multiplier is simply a number you multiply your BMR by to get your TDEE.

Activity Level	Multiplier	My Current BMR (Calories)	TDEE (Calories)
Sedentary (Little to no exercise, desk job)	1.2	1,932	2,318
Lightly Active (Light Exercise 1-3 days/week)	1.375	1,932	2,657
Moderately Active (Moderate Exercise 6-7 days/week)	1.55	1,932	2,995
Very Active (Hard Exercise Every Day)	1.725	1,932	3,333
Extra Active (Hard Exercise 2 or More Times a Day)	1.9	1,932	3,671

I would rate my activity level at Moderately Active. I try to do some sort of exercise every day. With that activity level, my TDEE is 2,995 calories per day. That means that to lose two pounds per week, I need to eat 1,995 calories per day. Remember: to lose two pounds per week you must be at a 1,000-caloric deficit per day.

$$2,995-1,000 = 1,995 \ cal/day$$

Depending on your activity level and desired weight loss target, your calorie goal will change. I will include a table below with all my options for calorie goals.

Activity Level	Calorie Goal for 1lb/week loss (TDEE – 500)	Calorie Goal for 2lb/week loss (TDEE-1,000)
Sedentary (Little to no exercise, desk job)	1,818	1,318
Lightly Active (Light Exercise 1-3 days/week)	2,157	1,657
Moderately Active (Moderate Exercise 6-7 days/week)	2,495	1,995
Very Active (Hard Exercise Every Day)	2,833	2,333
Extra Active (Hard Exercise 2 or More Times a Day)	3,171	2,671

These caloric estimates are much better, right? This is why exercise plays an important role in weight loss. If you want to eat more calories per day while still losing weight, you must exercise.

MACROWHAT?

At the end of the day, if you are in a caloric deficit, you are going to lose weight. However, you need to make sure you are giving your body the right nutrients. You can't eat doughnuts until you hit your calorie goal. Sure, that sounds delicious and you will lose weight if you remain at a caloric deficit, but it's not healthy and you're going feel miserable.

Roughly estimating, a doughnut is around 250 calories. If I eat seven doughnuts, I would be just under my calorie goal of 1,995 calories with 1,750 calories for the day. From experience, eating seven doughnuts is miserable. I don't know if it was really exactly seven doughnuts, but let me tell you a story.

I took a trip to Vegas with my friends. Now that I think about it, calories eaten in Vegas should have stayed in Vegas, but they did not. We decided to go to a doughnut shop for breakfast. After a night of questionable decisions, what's one more? We arrived at The Donut Bar and they all looked so good. We ended up with 10 doughnuts but the cashier told us that if we bought a dozen that we would get another doughnut for free. Obviously, we walked out of there with 13 doughnuts. Between the three of us, we each ate around 4.3 doughnuts. However, I forgot to mention, these weren't regular doughnuts. They had to have been double, maybe even triple, the size of a regular doughnut. So it's safe to assume I consumed the equivalent of seven doughnuts. Once I finished my share, I immediately regretted my decision. Not only did I feel sick, but I also felt hungry. Even though I met my calorie goal, I did not give my body the right nutrients to feel full and satisfied.

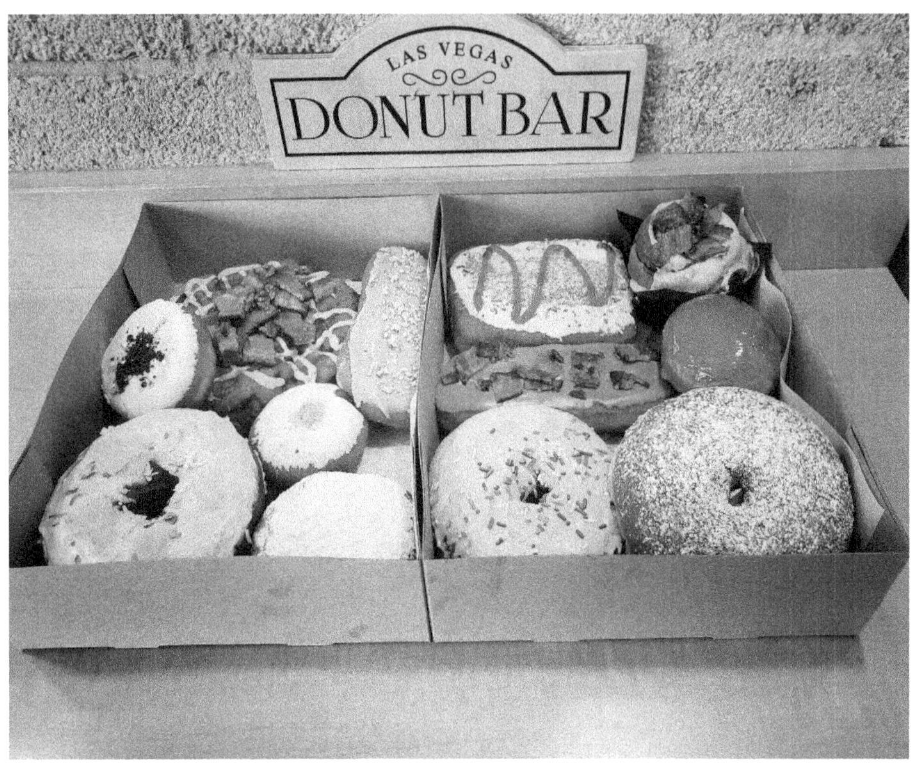
LAS VEGAS
DONUT BAR

There are two types of nutrients. Nutrients that your body requires a large amount of, called macronutrients, and nutrients that your body requires a smaller amount of, called micronutrients. I am going to focus on macronutrients or more commonly referred to as macros. Macros consist of proteins, carbohydrates, and fats. Proteins help build or maintain muscle among other things. Carbs provide energy for your brain and provide energy to your muscles while conserving muscle mass during exercise. Fats protect our vital organs, store energy, provide insulation, and help perform other biological functions.

Everything you consume is made up of macronutrients and can be any combination of the three. Carbs and protein have four calories per gram while fat has nine calories per gram.

The Institute of Medicine of the National Academies recommends 45-65% of calories from your DIEt should come from carbs, 20-35% from fats, and 10-35% from proteins based on their Acceptable Macronutrient Distribution Ranges (AMDR). I will show you how to calculate your macros based on the AMDR.

We're on the last bit of math here.

Remember, you won't have to worry about calculations. Everything will be done for you. I just want to explain where these numbers come from, so no need to panic.

For my DIEt, I prefer 45% carbs, 35% protein, and 20% fats. The numbers will be based on the TDEE calorie goal I calculated of 1,995 calories.

1,995 x .45 = 897.75 calories from carbs

1,995 x .35 = 698.25 calories from protein

1,995 x .20 = 399 calories from fat

Okay, so 897.75 of the calories I consume should come from carbs, 698.25 calories from protein, and the remaining 399 calories from fat. The percentages should add up to 100%. Next, I must change the calories to grams using the table provided below.

Calories Per Gram	
Protein	4
Carbs	4
Fats	9

*(897.75 cal of carbs) / (4 cal/gram) =
224.4375 grams of carbs*

*(698.25 cal of protein) / (4 cal/gram) =
174.5625 grams of protein*

(399 cal of fats) / (9 cal/gram) = 44.333 grams of fats

Now that I determined how many grams of each macronutrient I need to consume, I can calculate percentages.

224.4375 + 174.5625 + 44.333 = 443.333 total grams

*(224.4375 grams of carbs/ 443.333
grams) x 100 = 50% carbs*

*(174.5625 grams of protein/ 443.333
grams) x 100 = 40% protein*

(44.333 grams of fats/ 443.333 grams) x 100 = 10% fats

These are the macros I should be eating according to the ranges I picked from the AMDR. Whichever distribution of macronutrients you choose will not have a huge impact on weight loss because a calorie deficit is the KEY to weight loss. However, picking the right range of macros will make it easier for you to stick with your DIEt.

Now that you know the science of weight loss, I can show you how I did it. But first, I need to talk about DIEts.

DIET

Did you notice my spelling of the word, "DIEt?" I hope so.

If you have not, I am going to need you to focus a little more. I write my first book and you're not even paying attention!

One of the things a nutritionist said to me that I will never forget is "we don't use the word 'DIEt' because DIEt has the word,"DIE" in it and being in a DIEt for long periods of time makes you wanna DIE."

All DIEts work, for the most part, because they are all based on keeping your body at a caloric deficit. However, most aren't designed to be followed forever and none of them are personalized. You don't want to be on a DIEt your whole life, am I right? What usually ends up happening is you endure the DIEt for a couple of days, maybe a couple of weeks, only to end up back at the starting line. That's exactly what would happen to me.

What you must understand is to successfully lose weight and keep it off, going on a DIEt is not going to cut it. Instead, you must make the necessary changes to your eating habits that will change your lifestyle.

Not a DIEt change, a **lifestyle** change.

HOW I DID IT

Like I said before, losing weight is not magic; it's just science. Now that we understand the science, I can explain what I did to lose weight.

Thankfully, we have the technology to calculate your calorie goals and macros. Just grab your smartphone and download an app.

I'm not sure I can safely use the name of the app in my book, but the app I use starts with the word "my," includes the word "fitness" somewhere in there, and ends with the word "pal."

You can use any app you prefer. I'm sure other apps work just as well. There are free or paid versions of the app, but it's worth noting I succeeded with a free version.

Apps calculate your daily calorie limit. You'll need to log everything you eat on the app, and it will show you how many calories you are eating. It's tedious, I know, but you will get used to it after a while. Over time, you'll also start to learn more or less the number of calories you are eating, so don't worry. You won't be doing it forever.

Once you make an account and input your gender, age, weight, height, activity level, and weight loss goals, it will display your daily calorie goal. Note: the calories remaining estimate in this particular app is not your BMR or TDEE. It's your TDEE minus the caloric deficit corresponding to the number of pounds you want to lose per week. Once again, BMR stands for Basal Metabolic Rate. It is the number of calories you must consume for your body to perform it's basic functions to stay alive assuming you do not partake in any physical activity. TDEE stands for Total Daily Energy Expenditure and it is the amount of calories you burn when taking your activity level into consideration. As mentioned before, to lose one pound of fat, you must average a daily caloric deficit of 500 calories and 1,000 caloric deficit for two pounds per week.

With an app, you don't have to calculate anything. Just stick to the calorie goals the app gives you. I will include a table below showing the calorie goal numbers the app gives me so you can compare them to the calorie goals from my calculations. If you skipped the math chapter, just assume it's magic and go with the flow.

Activity Level Based on App	Calorie Goal Given by App
Not Very Active	1,500
Lightly Active	1,560
Active	1,920
Very Active	2,290

As you can see, the app does not provide the BMR or TDEE. It automatically gives you your daily calorie goals to follow. On my app profile, I selected "active" as my activity level, and I chose to lose two pounds of fat per week. The app tells me my daily calorie goal is 1,920 to reach my goal weight. The daily calorie goal I calculated was 1,995. The values are a little off, but that's normal because we do not know what equations they used to find the BMR and TDEE. Those small differences don't matter, so I stick with this number.

Every time you update your weight, the app will give you a new daily calorie goal. I recommend only checking your weight once a week on the same day around the same time, preferably early in the morning.

I found the app to be self-explanatory, so it should be easy to log what you're eating. The app keeps a database of almost every food you can imagine. Type in the name of the food in the data base or scan the barcode of what you are eating. There are rare occasions when specialty foods won't be available, so find something similar or manually input the nutritional values.

To accurately keep track of the calories you're eating, you'll need to buy a food scale. If you do not have a scale, you can estimate serving sizes, but to get the desired results you need to accurately measure the calories you're consuming. Do not cheat yourself; it's super easy to "estimate" one serving size when you're eating two.

Initially, I got away with estimating serving sizes. I was so overweight that reducing my portions to estimated serving sizes worked. However, if I had to start over, I would use a scale and measure my food from the beginning.

The serving sizes on the app are given in units of weight (ounces, grams, etc.), units of volume (cups, milliliters, etc.), or even as an item as a whole (1 protein bar, 1 cookie, 1 banana, etc.). All you have to do is measure out your food and input what you are eating. I will give you an example.

Search for "T-Bone steak" in the app. The serving size is automatically set to 4 ounces. But say you measure your steak to be 6 ounces. You have two options, input that you ate 1.5 servings, 1.5X4=6, or change the serving size to 1 ounce and input you ate 6 servings. Either way works, just make sure you input what you are eating correctly so that the calories consumed will be as accurate as possible. By the way, you weigh the steak after it is cooked not before. Same goes for all other protein.

A majority of the time, you'll consume one serving size of each food. That's how you're supposed to eat. There are food items you can afford to eat bigger serving sizes, like most vegetables, because their caloric impact is small. Be careful though. Starchy vegetables like potatoes and corn will act more as carbs and require smaller servings. If you use oil to cook vegetables, you're going to be eating more calories than steamed vegetables, so make sure you measure how much oil you use to cook your meals.

You're still eating the calories you don't keep track of, and they will add up throughout the day so try to be accurate. Again, don't cheat yourself! Logging you ate only one cookie when you ate three is not going to help you. Be honest with yourself and log EVERYTHING you eat.

Allow me to share a trick that helped me when I craved junk food. I would log it before I ate it. Often, I would immediately regret my decision and not eat it after seeing how many calories I was going to waste on a small snack.

Let's do a fun experiment. I want you to open up the app and log the food you have eaten for the past 3 days. If your memory isn't that great, log what you ate today or yesterday. Estimate the serving sizes, and if you're unsure, go ahead and log two serving sizes. By how many calories did you exceed your limit? 100? 1,000? 2,000?

The point of that experiment was to make you aware of the massive amount of calories you are consuming and where they are coming from. If you have been eating well and didn't exceed your limit, you are already on your way to weight loss.

Here are a couple of my daily meal entries to give you some examples.

Day 1	
Calorie Goal = 2,250	
Calories	**Breakfast**
120	Bread (2 Slices)
140	2 Eggs
105	1 Banana(126 grams)
	Snack
320	Jamba Juice (Small)
	Lunch
120	Pork Loin (4 Ounces)
16	1 Cucumber (133 grams)
215	Rice (1cup)
	Snack
90	Almonds (15 grams)
	Dinner
560	Stuffed Salmon with Broccoli (pre-made tray)
180	1 Sweet Potato
	Snack
160	1 Protein Shake
Total Cal	**Goal-Cal Consumed**
2026	**2,250-2,026=224 calories remaining**

Day 2	
Calorie Goal = 1,920	
Calories	**Breakfast**
160	1 protein shake
	Lunch
850	Fast Food Sandwich
	Dinner
330	1 Chicken breast (8 Ounces)
205	Rice (1 Cup)
	Snack
260	1 Lunchables
Total Cal	**Goal-Cal Consumed**
1805	1,920-1,805=115 calories remaining

I want to point out a couple of things from my two daily entries.

My calorie goal is different for these two days. I picked two dates a couple of months apart. As your weight goes down your calorie goal will start to change.

The day with more food entries (day 1), I ate healthier meals, so I was able to eat more food. It is recommended to eat something every three hours so you won't be starving between meals. This approach allows for three meals accompanied with three snacks.

The day with fewer entries (day 2), I ate at a fast-food restaurant for one meal, so I had to reduce the number of snacks to remain under my calorie limit. It's important to note, you can still eat out if you make the necessary adjustments.

For both samples, I was slightly under my calorie limit for the day. It's perfectly fine to reach your calorie limit, but you'll often find that you can eat a little less and be satisfied. This will aid in faster weight loss.

What you CANNOT do is go extreme and be way under your calorie goal. Remember, your calorie goal provided by the app is the recommended limit to lose weight at a healthy, sustainable rate. It's not healthy to be at an extreme caloric deficit. Your body will think it's starving and store the next meal you eat as fat instead of burning it off as energy.

Let me show you the extremes. We know that **weight loss = caloric deficit.** So technically, you can eat the meals I am about to show you and still lose weight.

Day 3	
Calorie Goal = 1,920	
Calories	Lunch
490	1 Large Fries
790	Burger
320	Large Soda
Total Cal	**Goal-Cal Consumed**
1600	**1,920-1,600=320 calories remaining**

Day 4	
Calorie Goal = 1,920	
Calories	**Snacks**
1820	7 Glazed Doughnuts
Total Cal	**Goal-Cal Consumed**
1820	**1,920-1,820=100calories remaining**

You are still going to lose weight, but you will be miserable with only one meal that day and you are not going to be hitting your macronutrients.

In case you skipped the math section, macronutrients are nutrients your body needs to perform as efficiently as possible. They consist of protein, carbs, and fats. The app magically calculates these numbers for you.

To find your macros on an iOS device, open your fitness app and select "Diary," scroll down and select "Nutrition." You can change these numbers if you wish by selecting "More," scrolling down and selecting, "Calorie, Carbs, Protein and Fat Goals."

To find your macros on an Android device, select "Diary." In the top right corner of the screen, select the pie chart then select, "Macros." You can change these numbers by selecting "Me," then selecting "Goals," scrolling down and selecting "Calorie, Carbs, Protein and Fat Goals."

In the beginning, I would suggest sticking with the macro percentages the app gives you. Remember that calorie deficit is the key to weight loss, but sticking with a healthy range of macronutrients will make the transition to your new lifestyle easier. If you eat nutritious food, you tend to be able to eat more meals throughout the day. If you eat junk, you will hit your calorie goal faster with less food. Remember that the acceptable macronutrient distribution ranges are 45-65% of calories from carbs, 20-35% from fats, and 10-35% from proteins.

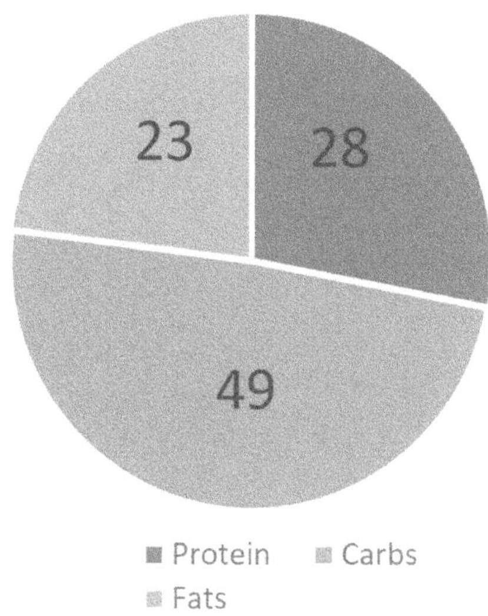

Day 1 Macronutrient Percentages
23
28
49
Protein   Carbs
Fats

Day 2 Macronutrient Percentages

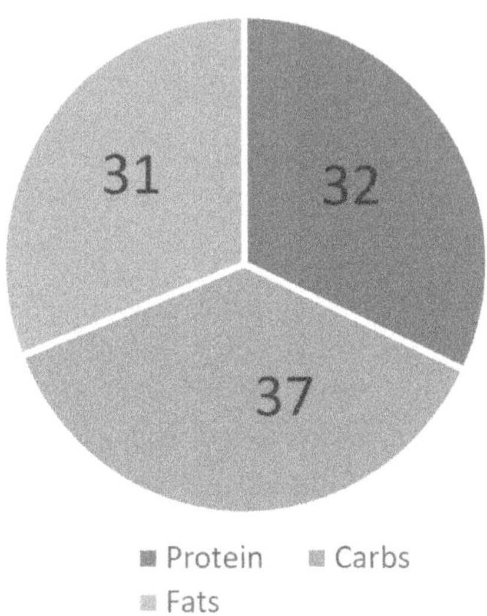

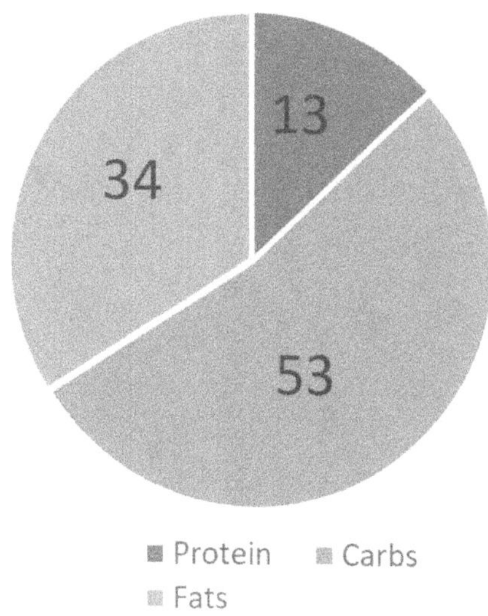
Day 3 Macronutrient Percentages
13
34
53
Protein
Carbs
Fats

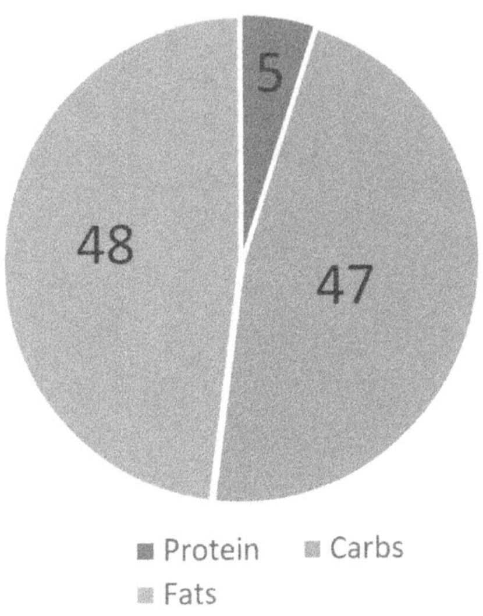

Day 4 Macronutrient Percentages
5
48
47
Protein
Carbs
Fats

Above, you'll see the macronutrient representation from four of my meals. As you can see, my healthiest day, day 1, is closest to the acceptable macronutrient range. The percentages start falling out of the acceptable range as the quality of meals decreases.

To hit your calorie goal and macros, it's going to be a lot of trial and error. You can use the meals I provided as an example, but don't worry if you're not hitting your goal at first.

I am not providing more daily meal examples because I am not a nutritionist. Besides, everybody's food preferences are different. You might not even like the things that I like to eat, which would be weird because I like to eat literally everything. More importantly, because you need to learn how to lose weight by yourself. I would recommend going to a nutritionist if you need someone to keep you accountable and give you guidance. However, you do not need someone to control YOUr DIEt and tell you exactly what to eat. Logging your food will give you the freedom to eat anything you want. Remember, as long as you are in a caloric deficit you will lose weight.

Begin this process by constantly logging EVERYTHING you eat so you can learn your calorie and nutrient consumption. Slowly start making the necessary changes to hit your calorie and macro goals. I know it's tedious, but this was the only way I was able to lose weight and keep it off. Trust me. It's worth it.

THE 1,000 CALORIE SALAD

A 1,000-calorie salad? I thought salads were supposed to be healthy? Sadly, any healthy meal can become unhealthy. If you don't pay attention to what you're putting in your salad, you can easily consume over 1,000 calories. If you start adding bacon, croutons, cheese, nuts, or dressing the calories will quickly add up. A peanut butter and jelly sandwich is another great example. PB&Js are easy, quick snacks to make. However, if you do not measure the correct serving size for peanut butter, you can easily ingest hundreds of calories.

Be conscious of what you are eating. Take everything into consideration.

<u>BYOB</u>

Guess what. Beer, wine, energy drinks, soda, and almost every drink other than water has calories. I don't drink alcohol so it was not something I have to worry about. You don't need to give up drinking. Just be aware that you'll need to fit them into your calorie goal.

Drinking calories is practically useless and it is one of the easiest ways to exceed your calorie daily limit. If you have room for them, go ahead. But think about it, if you are struggling with hunger you are going to want to save as many calories as possible for actual meaningful meals or snacks to keep you full and satisfied.

There are exceptions of course. Protein shakes or meal replacement drinks are a good healthy way to drink calories. Often times they will not leave you fully satisfied but they can be used as convenient meals or snacks if you do not have time to cook or have some left over calories at the end of the day.

The only other thing I would recommend drinking is water. Likely, you are not drinking enough water throughout the day. Drinking enough water is important to keep your body functioning properly. Regarding weight loss, drinking water can suppress your hunger.

Drinking a glass of water before every meal helps you feel more satisfied. Sometimes we cannot differentiate between hunger and thirst. When in doubt drink some water.

Again, log EVERYTHING do not leave out the calories you drink.

SCALE

We're usually obsessed with bodyweight. I know I was, and honestly, I still am sometimes. However, bodyweight is not a good estimate of progress. If you're working out, you are likely building muscle. Muscle weighs more than fat. If the number on the scale does not move, or even if it goes up, do not worry. Instead, pay attention to how your clothes feel and how you feel. Some scales can tell you your body composition, body fat percentage, muscle mass, bone mass, and even BMR. If you do not have one, as long as you have been at a caloric deficit, just keep going. There have been several times the number on my scale would not budge. One time it happened for three weeks, but I felt better and my clothes fit better. It was frustrating and hard to ignore, but just remember that the number on the scale does not always accurately represent your improvement or level of fitness. If you suddenly stop working out and stop watching what you eat, you can lose muscle and gain fat. In this case, the number on the scale might not move up, but your body composition will deteriorate. The best thing to do is just remain consistent no matter what the scale says. The results will come.

CONSISTENCY

To reiterate, what you eat is the most important factor in weight loss. All you have to do is remain consistent. It will take some time, but if you stick with it, you will see results. Consistency is a major factor in how quickly you'll be able to lose weight.

PEER PRESSURE

"What's one bad meal?" "Oh c'mon! Just start your DIEt again on Monday." I have been a victim of these types of phrases around a million times. I would be doing really well until someone invited me out to eat. From my experience, eating poorly for one day sets me back a whole week. Even so, it's difficult to say no. Here's another story.

I met up with two of my friends at one of their apartments. We were going to go workout together at the recreational center. Suddenly, we start talking about this burger place and how good it is. One of them says, "Screw it. Let's go eat there and start working out tomorrow?" Next thing you know, we're cruising down the road on our way for some burgers. On the way, there's a Krispy Kreme and, of course, the doughnut bat signal was on. (For those who don't know, Krispy Kreme places this sign outside of their store, kind of like a doughnut bat signal, that turns on every time they make a fresh batch of doughnuts. If you are lucky enough to walk in the store when the light is on, you get a free glazed doughnut. If you have never been, a fresh glazed doughnut from Krispy Kreme is amazing.) Back to the story, the light was on, and it was an opportunity we couldn't pass up. Walk in, grab our free doughnut, and walk out. One of my friends always feels bad just grabbing the free doughnut, so we end up leaving with half a dozen. We resume our trip to the burger place after each of us ate three doughnuts. The last obstacle remaining between us and a burger is this Italian shaved ice place. We had already made the drive. We had no choice but to stop there, too. We finally arrive at our initial destination, with several hundred more unplanned calories, and eat the burgers.

As you can tell, it does not take much to persuade me. It's always going to be tempting to give in to peer pressure, but here are some tips to help you evade it. First, you must change your mindset that you CANNOT eat something because you can. You are just making the CHOICE to eat or not eat certain things. It's much easier to think "I can eat a pizza, but I do not want to." Rather than think, "Damn, I can't eat pizza." Use the same principle when someone offers you food. Instead of saying "No, thanks. I can't." say "No thanks, I already ate." If you know you are going to be away from home, plan and take some snacks. If you go out to eat at a restaurant, there are tons of healthy options. Most menus list the calories per meal. If they don't, you can look them up on the app.

HOW MANY FATS DID I BURN?

Where does all the fat magically go? Turns out, again, it's not magic, it's science. There's this law called the Conservation of Mass that states "Matter cannot be created nor destroyed." Fat does not just disappear. It undergoes a chemical reaction and gets transformed into carbon dioxide and water molecules.

$$C_5 H_{104} O_6 + 78 O_2 \rightarrow 55 CO_2 + 52 H_2O$$

I never liked chemistry, so I'm not going to bore you with a detailed explanation. In simple terms, the equation says a fat molecule ($C_5 H_{104} O_6$) plus oxygen (O_2) will yield to carbon dioxide (CO_2) plus water (H_2O). Technically the more you breathe out, the more fat you burn.

Exercise plays a big role in losing weight. The more active you are, the more energy you use. But I want you to remember that what you eat is the most important aspect of weight loss. You can exercise all you want, but if you are not on a caloric deficit, you are not going to lose weight.

Make sure you are honest in choosing your activity

level on My Fitness Pal. The app increases your caloric intake depending on how active you are. If you select very active and are sedentary, you won't be at a caloric deficit.

If you have a smartwatch that tracks how many calories you burn daily, **DO NOT** add those burned calories to your daily calorie goal. The app is already accounting for those calories based on the activity level you chose.

You can try any type of workout you want, but you will never see results if you are not consistent.

CARDIO

This is what a typical run used to look like for me. I would start running until it was a bit uncomfortable and try to maintain that speed as long as possible. It usually never lasted more than a couple of minutes. I would have to walk until I caught my breath and start again. I repeated this until I was too tired to continue, which was usually around one mile. Not only would I get tired almost immediately, but I would also get knee pain, shin splints, you name it. Running sucked. It was exhausting and painful. I did not understand how people were able to run long distances while making it seem so easy. What was I doing wrong? Finally, I discovered the secret when I signed up for a marathon training class; monitoring your heart rate.

There are five heart rate zones based on your Max Heart Rate. To get a rough estimate of your MHR, you can use the Fox formula. Oops, I lied. This is the last bit of math.

$$220 - Age = MHR$$

Zone 1: 50-60% of MHR

This is an easy-effort zone used for warm-up and recovery.

Zone 2: 60-70% of MHR

Still at a comfortable pace, you should be able to maintain a conversation in this zone. This zone is typically labeled as the fat-burning zone. However, training above or below this zone will still yield fat loss. It is called the fat burning zone because your body mainly uses fat for energy in this heart rate range. At higher heart rate zones, the percentage of total used energy shifts from mainly using fats, to a combination of fats and carbs, to mainly using carbs. Remember that weight loss equals a caloric deficit. Exercising at any heart rate zone will help you be in a caloric deficit. However, exercising at this heart rate will train your body to use fat more efficiently.

Zone 3: 70-80% of MHR

This is the aerobic zone. In this zone, your body is still able to use oxygen to burn fat and use it as energy, but it also starts using carbs stored in your muscles as another source of energy. Training in this zone strengthens your heart, lungs, and teaches your body to manage and distribute oxygen more efficiently. It should feel like a moderate but comfortable pace that you can maintain for a long distance.

Zone 4: 80-90% of MHR

This is the anaerobic zone. Anaerobic exercise is an intense activity in which your body needs more oxygen than what your body can provide. Your body starts breaking down carbs stored in your muscles to use as energy instead of using oxygen. High-intensity efforts can only be maintained for a short period.

Zone 5: 90-100% of MHR

The final zone is when you train at your maximum effort. Training in this zone increases endurance, speed, and overall training capacity and it cannot be maintained for a long period of time.

Calories burned per hour will differ depending on the zone you are training on. You will burn the least amount of calories per hour training in zone 1 and you will burn the most amount of calories per hour training in zone 5.

Based on these training zones, you can perform steady-state cardio or high-intensity interval training. Steady-state cardio is an exercise in which you maintain the same speed for long periods, and it falls within training zones one to three. Some advantages of steady-state cardio include that your body's ability to use fat as energy increases, your endurance will increase, faster recovery times, and less stress on the body. Some disadvantages include extended workouts to burn significant calories and some people think it is boring. High-intensity interval training (HIIT)is an anaerobic exercise in which you perform shorter periods of intense effort, and it falls within training zones four and five. The main advantage HIIT holds over steady-state cardio is that you burn more calories in less time. However, it's an intense exercise that will push past your comfort zone and have more impact on the body. If your body is not prepared for this type of exercise, it can also cause more injuries.

Ideally, you should do a combination of both exercises. Steady-state helps you build endurance while HIIT helps you build strength, power, and speed.

I recommend beginning with steady-state cardio. It does not have to be running. You can go for a bike ride, swim, elliptical, or whatever you want. You might even reach zone two or three with a brisk walk.

If you don't have a smartwatch or a way to track your heart rate, I would strongly suggest buying one. You don't need to spend a crazy amount of money on one either. As long as it tracks your heart rate, you will be good. As your fitness level increases you will need a more accurate heart rate reading. At that point, you can consider investing in a more accurate heart rate monitor because being one beat per minute off could impact your training. But as a beginner any way to track your heart rate will suffice.

During your steady-state activity, find a comfortable pace that falls between zones one and three and maintain that speed for the duration of your workout. Do not worry about distance or pace. Focus on your duration of the runs. Your body doesn't know pace; it can only tell how much time you spend on your feet. Your endurance will improve over time. This is why long-distance runners can run so fast while making it seem effortless. Even though they're running fast, their heart rate is low. You have to be patient. It will take some time, but you will improve. When I first started training for a marathon, my comfortable pace was around 14 minutes per mile, and my heart rate hovered around 170bpm. Six months after I completed a marathon, my comfortable pace is 8:52 minutes per mile with my average heart rate at 165bpm. I did not understand the importance of building up your aerobic base until recently. I didn't use heart rate zones while marathon training. My focus at the time was to keep my heart rate under 170bpm. I still improved. However, I believe I would have made better progress if I had built a better aerobic base.

For the last couple of months I have been using the Maffetone method to train. Essentially it is a training method that forces you to keep your heart rate at zone 3 or below. I have noticed improvements in the three months that I have used this method. When I started training with this method, my pace was 13 minutes per mile in order to stay at zone 3 or below. For me, to remain in zone 3 I cannot exceed 153 beats per minute. After 3 months my pace has improved to 10.5 minutes per mile. Using this method I managed to improve my pace by almost a full 3 minutes while remaining within zone 3. At zone 3 I feel like I can run forever, and that is the idea of this training method. Improving your pace while keeping your effort (heart rate) the same. This is how you build your aerobic base.

To sum it up, steady-state cardio is used to build an aerobic base (zone three or below) but burns fewer calories over time. HIIT (zone four and five) is used to gain strength and speed and burn more calories in less time. Both work for weight loss, so I recommend doing both. I run four times a week; three of those runs are SSC and one is HIIT.

WEIGHT TRAINING

Weight training is important for weight loss. The more muscle you have, the more calories your body burns while at rest. There are tons of other health benefits that accompany putting on some muscle mass. Everyday tasks, like taking groceries from your car to your house in one trip, become easier. Nagging injuries and aches disappear. You will feel and look better. I wish I would have taken weight training more seriously when I was at higher fat percentages. I was never consistent enough. Even though I noticed improvements in strength, I never noticed much muscle definition. As your body fat percentage drops you will start to notice the improvements in your physique.

Consuming enough protein is important to build muscle. Studies show you need to intake at least 0.73 grams of protein per pound of body weight. Some even recommend intaking as much as 1 gram of protein per pound of body weight. You will need to adjust your macros so you are consuming between 0.73-1.00 grams of protein per body weight. This simply means to multiply your body weight times the range provided. Adjust your app settings to include your protein goal. You don't need supplements to hit your protein goal you can get it all from your diet. If you intake more protein than your body can process, it's dumped out, wasted. If you cannot consume enough protein from your diet you should drink protein shakes, but again, they are not required.

What do we need to do to build muscle? When we partake in resistance training, like lifting weights, we create micro-tears in our muscles. When the muscle repairs, muscle mass is added. A bunch of science and magical stuff happens when muscles are repaired. Nutrition and sleep play a key role in this process.

There are essentially two different types of weight training, bodybuilding and strength training. Bodybuilding training is generally used to build muscle for aesthetic purposes, while strength training is simply used to gain strength without worrying about your looks. As a beginner, it does not matter what you do; you will notice improvements either way. You won't notice improvements in strength without bigger muscles and you won't notice bigger muscles without improvements in strength. Executing the lifts with proper form is the most important thing to focus on. As you become more experienced, you can then opt to train around your goals. For weight loss, it's recommended to focus more on compound exercises, exercises that focus on more than one muscle group, and full-body workouts.

It's tough to recommend a specific lifting program because it depends on what type of equipment you have available, what type of shape you are in, and even how many times per week you are willing to work out. I started by researching lifting programs on the internet and sticking with one. There are weight training programs for weight loss, strength training, etc. There are also programs based on your equipment. You can also make progress with body-weight exercises. Do not get discouraged if that is all you have. If you are completely lost and need more assistance, you can look for a personal trainer. This might be the best alternative if you are a complete beginner because they'll help you build a more personalized program. Some gyms give a few sessions for free with a personal trainer, which might be all you need to get started.

My advice is to be patient and remain consistent no matter what you choose to do. You will see the results. Any new type of workout will probably feel uncomfortable maybe even miserable at the beginning, but it gets better with time. Once you start seeing progress, it becomes addicting and you will enjoy working out. From my experience, the exercises that benefited me the most were pull-ups, squats, bench presses, and deadlifts. Remember: just showing up to the gym doesn't equal results. Be conscious of what you are doing. You're already there—might as well put in the effort. I found the key factors for gaining muscle are consistency and trying to get better every single workout. You need to focus on progressive overload, a gradual increase of stress on your muscles. If you demand more from your muscles, they will have no choice but to grow. Increasing the load you lift by even 5 pounds per week will make a tremendous difference. Lifting light weight repeatedly without challenging your body isn't going to get you anywhere.

HI. IS YOUR SLEEPING SCHEDULE MESSED UP?

Sleep is something that most people don't get enough of even though we should. Sleep is important for many reasons. Lack of sleep can increase your chances of chronic diseases. It will also hinder your ability to grow muscle and lower performance during your workouts and everyday activities. Sleep also plays a factor in weight loss.

Leptin and ghrelin are two hormones that are affected by how much sleep you get. Leptin essentially tells your body when you should stop eating, gives you the "I am full" feeling, and when it should start burning calories. Ghrelin, on the other hand, tells your body when to keep eating and when to store calories as energy or fat. Lack of sleep reduces leptin hormones and increases ghrelin hormones. Weight loss is already challenging enough—get more sleep!

INJURY PREVENTION

When I got down to around 240 pounds I started exercising more. After seeing the results achieved from food alone, I wanted to see what I could do if I added exercise. I was still in college and finally started using the recreation center consistently. I would go with two friends at least five times per week and we would spend anywhere from two to three hours at the rec. A little crazy, I know, but exercising was finally fun. It is so much easier to exercise at a lighter weight, and it gets addicting when you start seeing results. We would start by playing a couple of, "around the world" basketball games as a warm-up. Then we would lift weights. After, we would run for 30 minutes on the track. Finally, we would play a couple of games of racquetball. If the racquetball courts were taken, we would play pickup basketball games. It was so fun. I managed to get down to 198 pounds. Everything was going great. Suddenly, my right knee bothered me for a couple of months. One day, during a run, it felt a little weird. I was around the midpoint of my run when I noticed something wasn't right, but I decided to push through. After I got home and I started to cool down, my knee started to swell. It got so bad that I could not bend my knee at all. If I tried, it felt like it was going to blow up. After a couple of doctor visits, I was diagnosed with patellar tendonitis. The doctor said I could live with the pain forever or opt for surgery. I decided to get surgery. I wasn't able to exercise for six months, and I ended up regaining the weight I lost. Before I was cleared to return to normal activities, I went to physical therapy and learned I had weak glutes and hips from not activating them properly. Lack of glute activation commonly leads to knee injuries. Instead of your muscles handling the forces experienced during running and jumping, they all go to your knees. Tendonitis is usually developed from overuse. I had been working out more than ever and was not aware that I was not using the proper muscles to exercise safely and efficiently.

Injuries happen, and sometimes, they can't be avoided. However, if you ensure you're executing proper form and recruiting the proper muscles, your risk of injury reduces greatly. Learn how to execute proper form. There is tons of useful online information for almost any exercise. YouTube is a great resource with videos of trainers explaining proper form and what you should feel. You can also ask your friends or someone in the gym for help. After you perform an exercise, be aware of what muscles are sore. Did you work those muscles? Are they supposed to be sore, or why are they not sore? I will give you an example.

After the first five-kilometer (5k) race I ran, my quadriceps were my only sore muscles. I thought it was normal. After therapy and running a marathon, I quickly learned that it is not normal. Running involves more than just the quadriceps. It involves quads, glutes, hamstrings, hips, calves, core, and other smaller stabilizing muscles. My main issues were weak hips and glutes, lack of glute activation, and simply not knowing how to run. I can almost guarantee that you do not know how to properly run either. There is more to running than just putting one foot in front of the other. I cannot recommend anything specific to correct your running form because there are too many variables and everyone is different. Some common issues that affect running form are over-striding, weak glutes, tight hips, tight hamstrings, poor ankle mobility, etc. If you are going to be running, I strongly suggest fixing your form to avoid injuries. It's better to start off doing it right instead of building bad habits and trying to correct them later. Some videos show how to run properly, but getting help from an experienced runner helped me the most. There are specialty running stores, like Fleet Feet, that host free running clinics every so often.

The next thing I want to talk about is ego lifting. Everybody starts somewhere. Don't be embarrassed if you can only lift light weights. Don't let your ego get the best of you. You are going to make improvements, so there's no need to rush them. When you lift more weight than you can handle, your form will break down and you risk injuring yourself. The same goes for cardio. Don't run crazy distances without building up to them.

Fix your muscle imbalances and prevent creating new ones. A muscle imbalance occurs when opposing muscles are not equal in strength and flexibility.

They can be caused by exercising with bad form, daily repetitive activities, or inactivity of certain muscles. Imbalances put unnecessary stress in your joints and will cause injuries over time. In my case, I had a muscle imbalance that resulted in knee surgery. My glutes and hamstrings were not developed enough, so my quadriceps overpowered them in certain exercises. Moreover, my quadriceps were imbalanced, which caused the movement of my patella to be irregular. A lot of injuries can be prevented by correcting muscle imbalances. You might have developed muscle imbalances and you don't want to create more. To prevent creating more muscle imbalances, do not neglect any part of your body. Shoulder injuries are other common examples caused by muscle imbalances. We tend to focus on exercises that strengthen the front part of the shoulder and neglect the muscles in the back. This then yields shoulder pain and injuries.

Using the right equipment designed for the activity you are doing will also help lower your risk of injury. Think about it, you are not going to play basketball with soccer cleats, right? It just doesn't make sense. It's the same principle for running and lifting weights. It is not recommended to use running shoes for lifting heavy weight or weightlifting shoes for running. I stumbled across Fleet Feet after knee surgery when I wanted to get fitted with the proper running shoes. They take a 3D scan of your foot and analyze how you walk and run, then they help you determine the best shoe for you. They can also give you tips and tricks for more enjoyable and efficient runs. I got fitted with one of my friends that trained for the marathon with me. Turns out that he had been wearing the wrong running shoe size all his life and did not know it. His feet would always bother him on long runs and he never understood why. There are even special socks for running. Cotton socks tend to create friction between your foot and your shoe which causes blisters. Running with blisters is not fun. If you experience chafing, there are products to prevent that as well.

Flexibility is also crucial in preventing injuries. A lack of flexibility can prevent you from performing exercises properly and even cause muscle imbalances.

Rest and recovery are crucial in avoiding injuries. During exercise your body breaks down and you need to rest to allow it to recover. Without proper recovery you will never reach your true potential. Recovery includes stretching, sleeping, and eating properly to fuel your body.

In summary, don't just jump into an exercise blindly with no experience. There is a right way to do everything. Do a little research, ask for help, and most importantly, listen to your body. If something does not feel right, try to figure out why. Do not let small nagging pains turn into bigger injuries.

MOTIVATION

After my knee surgery, I hovered around 230 pounds for a while. I got complacent. I was not happy with my weight. I knew that I could start losing more weight whenever I wanted to, but why did it take me so long to restart? I had a lack of motivation.

Then one day out of the blue, my dad got a message from a relative we had not seen in years. It was from his uncle. He told my dad that they were going to be in town because one of his daughters had a competition coming up and wanted to know if we were available. To me, at the time, they were strangers. I had not seen my dad's uncle since I was around five years old, and I had never met his daughters. I knew of them but never talked to them and wasn't sure if they knew who I was. Anyway, I finally got to meet my dad's uncle, aunt, and one of his cousins. The other cousin traveled with her team, so I didn't get to meet her until the competition. She competed in Modern Pentathlon. Have you ever heard of it? Yeah, me either. It's an Olympic sport in which you compete in five different events: fencing, freestyle swimming, equestrian show jumping, and a final combined event of pistol shooting and cross country running. The first time I saw her, she was decked out in her fencing gear and was warming up. I said hello and proceeded to the bleachers to watch the competition. I had no idea what was going on, but let me tell you, fencing is a fun event to witness in person. Luckily, her older sister competed before and explained all the rules and some strategies. She ended up placing in second for the individual event and won first place for the relay event. Until it was all over, I had no idea of the importance of that competition. She competed in the Youth Pan American Championships, which featured athletes from Guatemala, the Dominican Republic, Mexico, Canada, Argentina, the United States, and others. Winners of these games moved on to compete in the Youth Olympics in Buenos Aires, Argentina. I'm not so sure how the qualification process works, but she had already qualified for the Youth Olympics and competed in them later that year. After the competition, I talked about my weight loss journey with her and told her I wanted to get back in the gym and get in better shape after watching her compete. Before she left, she asked me to promise that I would be in better shape by the next time we saw each other. I said yes.

I started counting calories and exercising again shortly after that. I wasn't motivated to work out on many occasions. Almost every time that happened, I would come across her stories on Instagram. Sometimes I would be waking up and I would see on her stories that she already worked out once and was getting ready for another workout. She helped me push through.

You need to find your motivation. Maybe you made a promise to someone. Maybe you are going through a breakup, or maybe you're trying to get the attention of someone you like. Whether you're trying to fit back into that one pair of jeans or finally ready to prove to yourself that you can do it, find something that will help you push through. There are going to be moments when you don't feel like exercising or when you want to eat that thing you have been craving. In those moments, remember why you are doing this in the first place and you will push through.

Another thing that helped me was signing up for races and events. The way I see it, you pay all this money to race; you might as well train for them. You don't want to show up and get annihilated.

Surrounding yourself with people that support you during your weight loss journey is also beneficial. You can do it alone, but having people supporting you along the way will make it easier and more enjoyable. Luckily, I have friends that have always willingly, I think, joined me in my adventures. Whether it'd be the Spartan Races, training for a marathon, or even running 10 miles on the weekends for no reason. There have been countless times when I did not feel like working out, but my friends were there to hold me accountable. Even if you do not have anyone to work out with, simply talking to someone can make a difference. Seeing others succeed around you should motivate you. If they can do it, so can you. You will also pick up better habits and knowledge if you surround yourself with more health-conscious people.

IS THIS SPARTA?

I had seen videos of obstacle races on social media and always thought that it would be cool to race and complete those obstacles. I always imagined that I would feel and look like a badass if I completed one of those races. However, I never thought I would be able to do one. My friend and I would always say we would sign up for one someday once we were in good enough shape.

One day, we finally purchased the Spartan Trifecta pass. The Spartan Trifecta pass includes three spartan races, the sprint, super, and beast. If you complete those three races in a calendar year, you complete the Spartan trifecta. The sprint is three or more miles of obstacle racing with 20 obstacles. The Spartan Super is 8 miles or more with 25 obstacles, and the Spartan Beast is 13 or more miles with 30 obstacles. The distances for the races are now standardized to 5k, 10k, and half-marathon distances. When I raced, the distances varied. If you fail an obstacle in the race, you have to do 30 burpees. The races were about two months apart from each other, so I had time to train for them. I did not think we were in good enough shape yet but I hoped they would help me train and get in better shape to complete them.

A little more than a month before the Sprint, I finally started training. I will admit, I should have started training way before, but I did not think I would have too much trouble with the first race. I watched some videos of races to see what the obstacles looked like. Immediately, I identified several obstacles that seemed challenging. There are a bunch of hanging obstacles that seemed intimidating. My upper body strength was not good. The next day I went to a park that has a third of a mile paved track with several obstacles. I wanted to practice the monkey bars and jumping over an 8-foot wall. If you would have been there that day, you would have witnessed me getting out of my car, jogging to the monkey bars, failing the monkey bars, walking in defeat back to my car, and driving off. I don't think I attempted to do monkey bars since I was a little kid, and yes, I failed then too. On my drive back home, I was plagued with self-doubt. There is no way I can do this. What was I thinking? I should have started training sooner. I am going to die at some point during the race. Why did I sign up for this dumb (insert your favorite combination of cuss words here) race?! But then, I realized this was exactly why I signed up for the races. I needed something to push me past my comfort zone. I knew that it was not going to be easy. When I got home, I researched tips on how to do monkey bars. I found a bunch of helpful information, even little things like how to grip the bar. I showed up to the same park the next day and redeemed myself. It was still difficult, but knowing an actual technique helped tremendously. I should have read more about gripping the bar. I tore the skin on my left hand from gripping the bars incorrectly, but it was another lesson learned. Next on the list was the most-intimidating obstacle—the 16-foot rope climb. I bought a rope so I could practice. I did not attach it to anything super high, but I was able to practice the technique. Race day finally came, and I think we did pretty well. Our time was not great, but I was happy that we completed the race. I failed five obstacles, so I had to do 150 burpees. However, I was able to do the monkey bars with ease, and I was able to climb the rope. The rope climb was by far the most challenging obstacle I completed in my opinion. The 16-foot rope seemed a lot higher than I expected. I practiced with the rope I purchased in perfect, dry conditions. My rope was also thicker, so it was easier to climb. The rope at the race was smaller, muddy, wet, and I honestly wasn't sure if I could do it. I started to climb the rope insecure and full of doubt. After reaching the top, and ringing the bell, I came back down full of pride and confidence. I was humbled after the first race. I learned that I needed more upper body strength, to give myself more time to train, that burpees sucked, but most importantly, that I could do it.

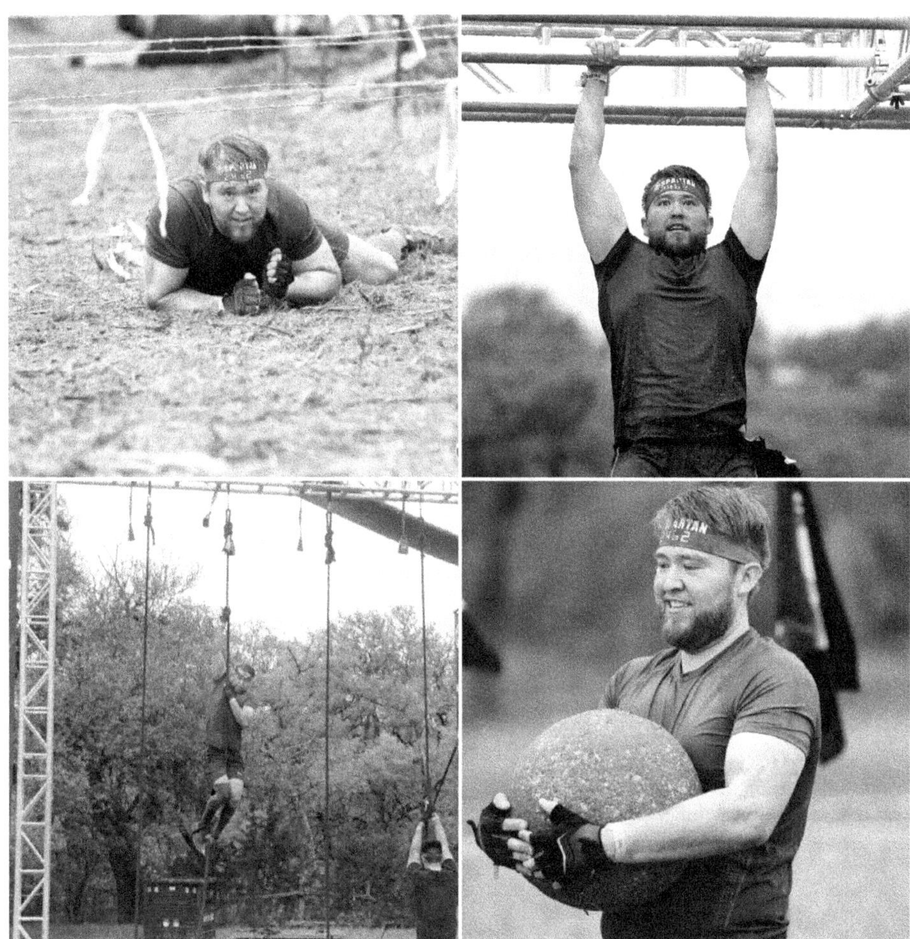

The Spartan Super was next. I trained more for this race than the first one. I was finally able to do my first pull up while training for this race. It was a big achievement for me. I never even got close to doing one single pull up. I completed more obstacles that required upper body strength in this race, but I was not prepared for the distance. The longest distance I ever ran up to this point was three miles, and this race was eight miles long. It seemed like we were cruising along until one of my friends started cramping around mile six. Funny story, as we were helping my friend stretch out on the side of the trail some guy stopped by and gave us a packet of mustard. He said, "Here, man. It will help with the cramps." We thanked him, but wondered "What the hell are we supposed to do with the mustard? Rub it on his leg?" This is before we were aware of how important nutrition was during races. He was supposed to eat the mustard to give his body some carbs for fuel. Thankfully, we did not rub the mustard on his leg and he ate it. We just did not know why. Not long after, I started cramping as well. It was a struggle from then on. We would have to stop occasionally to stretch. The worst for me was at the very end. There was a final hill that led up to the rope climb, which I had to stop for a couple of minutes to stretch my hamstrings. They were both cramping. It was pretty funny actually, well funny now and not then. I would get rid of the cramp on my hamstrings, then my quads would immediately cramp up. I did not know which was worse, so I just sort of embraced the pain until I was able to get to the rope climb. Obviously, I was not able to do the rope climb.

THIRTY BURPEES later, I still had one last obstacle to go. It is probably one of the easiest obstacles, but not when your muscles are cramping. The last obstacle was the A-frame, a 30-foot cargo net that you climb over. I remember pausing at the very top for "pictures" when really, I stopped to rest a little bit so I would not cramp on the way down. We finished the eight-mile race only a couple of minutes slower than the first race. We either performed poorly on the first race or made big improvements in the second race. I like to think that we improved. I only had to do 120 burpees that race. It was an improvement because I did less than the first race even though there were more obstacles. Once you finish the race, there is a big tent to change into clean clothes. I wasn't even able to take off my socks. As soon as I would reach down and make the effort to pull my socks off, I would start cramping. In my defense, they were knee-high compression socks that were stuck to my skin after running through dirt and mud for hours. Still, it should not have been that exhausting to take some socks off. It took me about 15 minutes to change. On the way back home, I started cramping everywhere. Even my non-existent abs started cramping. It was the worst I've ever felt. From the second race, I learned my upper-body training was working, but I needed to be able to run longer distances.

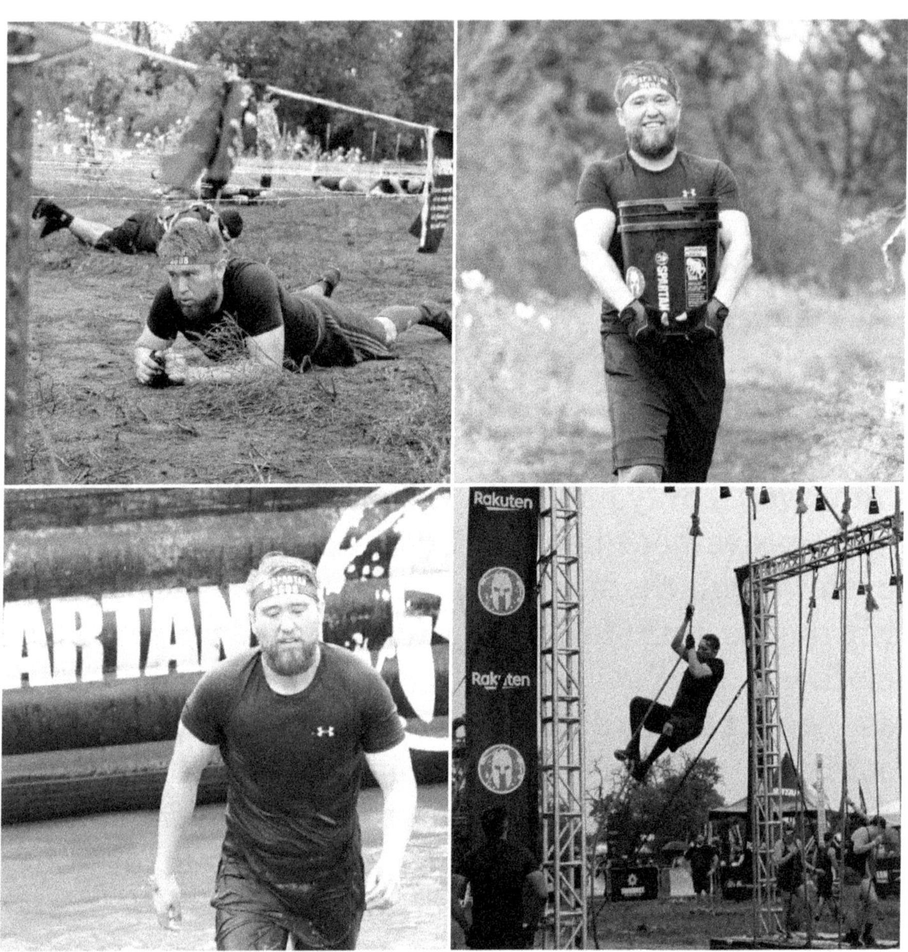

Two races down; one to go. Only the most challenging race remained to complete the trifecta, the Spartan Beast. I did not want to cramp like that again, so my friend and I signed up for a marathon class. The class perfectly aligned with the Beast. The weekend of the race was the same weekend our class would run 18 miles. During our marathon class, we learned about nutrition during a race. Your muscles will run out of energy during a long race, so it's recommended to refuel every 45 minutes so you can keep going. The last useful thing we learned was to pace ourselves. We learned what our comfortable running pace for long distances. We started too fast and did not refuel in the first two races, so by the end, we were running on fumes. Most likely, all these factors contributed to the cramping. Race day arrived and I felt prepared for it. We started slow and a bunch of people passed us. As the race went along, we started passing up almost everyone that passed us at the beginning of the race. Our preparation paid off. The course was tough, but I was able to complete almost all the obstacles. I only failed 2 obstacles, so I only had to do 60 burpees. Not bad at all.

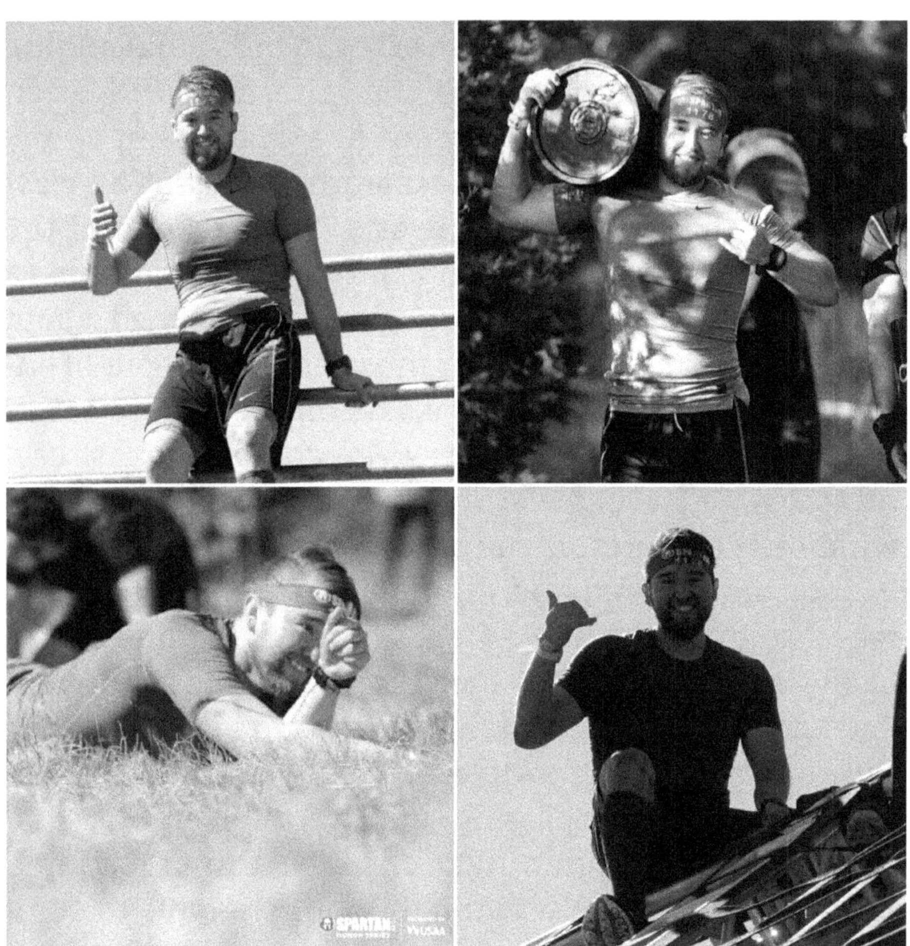

EASY, FUN THREE-MILE JOG

I had no idea what to expect on the first day of marathon training. I remember being nervous but eager to begin. All of a sudden, the coach walks out after introductions and says, "Today we are only doing a fun, easy three-mile jog." My friend and I immediately looked at each other in confusion. I thought to myself, "Fun? Easy? Three miles?" I never thought those words could be used in a coherent sentence.

All my life, I have despised running. As mentioned earlier, I was terrible at it. It was painful, it didn't make sense, it was my arch-nemesis. What in the world am I doing training for a marathon? I thought about this endlessly, but after cramping at the Spartan Race, I knew I had to try. I wanted to finally enjoy running, or at least not hate it, and most importantly finally be good at it.

I found out about the training when I went to get fitted for shoes at Fleet Feet. It was a 17-week training plan which consisted of runs on Monday, speed drills on Wednesdays, a run on Thursdays, and long runs on Saturdays. On average, we were running 27 miles per week. Including the marathon, I ran around 422 miles in 17 weeks. Before I started training, my longest run was at the Spartan Super, which was only 8 miles. After training for a while, I got to the point where running anything less than 10 miles felt super easy. Around halfway through the training program, I was breaking my distance record with every long run. My big achievements include running 10 miles for the first time, running the first half marathon (13.1 miles), running 15 miles, and running 20 miles. Of course, my most proud accomplishment was finishing the 26.2 miles of the marathon. I got a new personal record for my mile run at 6 minutes 20 seconds. For years, I wasn't able to run a mile under 14 minutes. This marathon class also introduced me to heart rate training and nutrition during the race. The first couple of weeks of training sucked. It was the most I ever ran in my life. After a while, I got used to it and it got easier. Plenty of people asked me why I was doing it, and some would tell me I was crazy for wanting to run a full marathon. Initially, the main motivation for marathon training was to be prepared for the Spartan Beast. I wasn't sure I would sign up for a marathon and didn't sign up until about a month before the race. Honestly, I didn't really have a reason to run the marathon and not even sure if I could do it.

Two weeks before the marathon, I got sick with the influenza. I had to stop training. I could not eat anything or drink much and just slept for that whole week. When I went to the doctor, she told me that I might not be able to run the marathon. It would just depend on how quickly my body got over the flu. I slowly started to feel better but was not fully there yet. Three days before the marathon, we had our last training session. It was an easy, fun 2.5-mile jog. It did not seem that fun or easy. It felt good to finally run again, but I did not like how 2.5-miles felt three days before I had to run 26.2 miles. I talked to my coach about it and he said as long as I felt able to run that I should be fine. One week of doing nothing was not going to ruin 16 weeks of training. The night before the marathon, I knew I was not 100% but there was no way I was not going to run. I started getting all my things ready for the next morning. Favorite running shirt, running shorts, running socks, compression shorts, running belt, running hat, running watch, anti-blister foot balm, race bib, and nutrition for the race. (I took eight energy gels, three Roctane Gus, five Huma energy gels, and one Honey Stinger Energy Waffle.) Everything was ready to go. I was ready. All I needed now was to get a good night's sleep. What is sleep? Who knows? I probably slept for three hours.

Race day. There were approximately 18,000 people registered for the Rock 'n' Roll San Antonio Marathon & Half Marathon. I struggled a bit to get to my corral, your designated area to start the race based on your estimated finishing time. Finally, it was time to start. The first couple of miles felt like the easiest miles I ever ran. I guess that's what the coach meant by easy, fun three-mile jog. I noticed several times I was going too fast. I was targeting an average pace of ten minutes per mile.

I caught myself going well under that, but it felt comfortable. The first half of the marathon was a breeze. I finished it in 2 hours and 6 minutes. Side note, Eliud Kipchoge broke the world record time for a full marathon in 2019. He finished it in 1 hour 59 minutes and 40 seconds. That is INSANE. His average pace was 4 minutes and 34 seconds per mile. But back to my story. Just before the halfway point the course split. Full marathoners went left, and half marathoners went right. I was surrounded by people for that first half, but once we split, I felt like I was running alone from mile 13 to mile 14. That's when I started feeling a little tired. I decided to walk for a bit to eat my Honey Stinger waffle. I can eat energy gels and drink water while running, but I cannot chew solid food and run. I walked for maybe 5 minutes as I finished my waffle. I was hungry and wanted to savor it as long as possible. As I walked, more people started showing up around me. So, I started running again. At mile 15, I spotted a port-a-potty and decided to make a pit stop. My legs were super stiff at this point, but the running continued. Suddenly, I started cramping. I slowed down, changed my stride, and kept going. At mile 16, I decided I needed to walk for a bit. From the Spartan races, I learned I could push through cramps for a while, but at a certain point, the cramping would get so bad that I would need to completely stop. I walked for a full hour. Occasionally, I would make an effort to run to see if I could but would have to stop. During this stretch, it seemed as if the majority of the 18,000 runners were passing me. I got angry, sad, and I even teared up a little bit. I thought all the training I did was for nothing. Maybe people were right. Maybe signing up for a marathon was crazy. Off in the distance, I started hearing some music. It was a song that became popular and played on the radio around the time I graduated from college. It instantly changed my mindset and mood. When I signed up for marathon training, I went into it thinking the main benefit was to prepare my body to run long distances, and it did. However, the most important thing that came out of it was helping me break through mental barriers. There were so many days when I did not want to go train and just give up in the middle of my run. Every new distance record, 5, 8, 10, 15, 20 miles, all seemed impossible. What was so different about 26.2 miles? I also started thinking about all the different people I encountered while running the marathon. Thousands of people cheering you on. The other runners, each with their unique story and purpose of running. But the ones that impacted me the most were the people in wheelchairs, the cancer survivors, and the people running for someone that couldn't or wasn't there anymore. I can't even imagine the things they have endured. What was my excuse? So, I started running again. I still felt as if cramping could come back so I would take small walking breaks. At mile 24, I decided that I would push through without stopping. What're two more miles? Finally, I could see the finish line. I probably had less than a fourth of a mile to go and wanted to stop so bad. I was about to stop for a bit so I could go all out on the final straightaway. Suddenly out of nowhere, one of my friends started running beside me. I have no idea where he came from. I didn't even know he was going to show up. "You are almost there. You got this. Your family is waiting at the finish line. I'm gonna go tell them you are about to finish." He said as he sprinted away. I did not stop. I started speeding up, or so I thought. Not sure if my legs allowed me to go any faster, but at least it felt like it. Every single step I took felt like I was going to cramp. Quads, hamstrings, calves, random leg muscles I didn't even know existed. To be honest, I don't know how I was able to run that last portion of the race. After 5 hours, 36 minutes, 17 seconds, and 4,529 calories, I was finished. I am not too happy with that time. I know I could have finished faster. I think getting sick did not help. I guess I am going to have to run another one to find out.

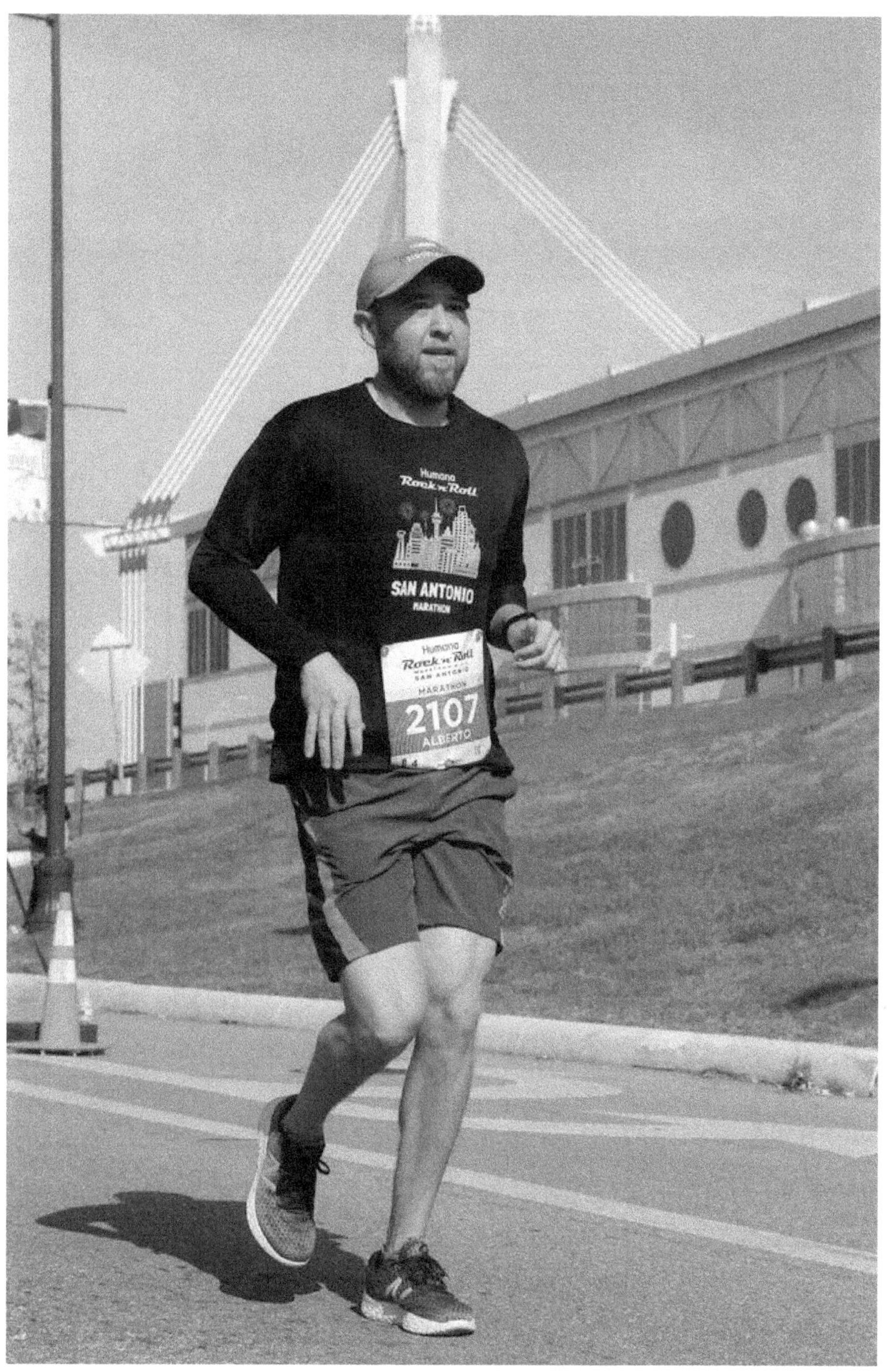
Humana
Rock 'n' Roll
SAN ANTONIO
MARATHON
Humana
Rock 'n' Roll
SAN ANTONIO
MARATHON
2107
ALBERTO

PROGRESS IS PROGRESS

It is human nature to always want something more. To seek to be better, faster, stronger, to lose weight quicker, etc. This is normal. Wanting better results is ultimately what drives us to accomplish our goals. However, we must take a step back every once in a while and look at how far we've come and be proud of everything we have accomplished during our journey no matter how insignificant it might seem. Even if it's merely your first push up, first pull-up, first time running a mile nonstop, losing one pound of fat, logging your food every day for a week, fitting into a smaller size, anything. Progress is Progress. Every challenge you overcome is proof that you are heading in the right direction. Daily "insignificant" victories add up, and ultimately, they are what will determine if you accomplish your goal or fail once again.

I am going to share with you one of my favorite quotes. It's a quote that has been hanging in the San Antonio Spurs locker room for a while now, but it resurfaced when they won the 2014 NBA Championship. After losing the 2013 championship, it still hurts talking about that, the Spurs came back and dismantled the Heat in five games while playing some of the most beautiful basketball all season long. If you don't agree with me on this, sorry to tell you, but you're wrong. Check out some highlights on YouTube. Anyway, the Spurs adopted their mentality "Keep pounding the rock" from this quote:

> *"When nothing seems to help, I go and look at a stonecutter hammering away at his rock perhaps a hundred times without as much as a crack showing in it. Yet at the hundred and first blow, it will split in two, and I know it was not that blow that did it, but all that had gone before." — Jacob Riis*

Focus on daily progress, get better every single day, and success will come.

NEWTON'S FIRST LAW OF MOTION

Sorry, I could not end the book without one last science reference. Newton's First Law of Motion states an object at rest stays at rest and an object in motion stays in motion unless acted upon by an external force. What does this have to do with weight loss? Well, nothing really. It's just an easy way for me to try to get my point across so that you'll remember it.

What I am trying to say is you are the object at rest. You will remain the same until you make the necessary changes, the external force. Once you get going, your weight loss will remain in motion unless acted upon by an external force, complacency.

Making that lifestyle change and consistently sticking to it is hard. Once you start seeing results and get used to the new routine, it's not as hard to keep going. If you reach your goal and are still not happy with the way you look or feel, immediately set a new goal and start working to accomplish it. Do not stop. The hardest part of weight loss and getting in shape is getting started. So why stop all that momentum? Just keep the ball rolling! If you become complacent and stop for whatever reason, it's going to be hard to start again.

CONCLUSION

During one of our final lectures, my Engineering Senior Design professor said, "The greatest thing we can take from getting an education is developing the ability to learn." I think part of the problem of why we struggle to change is because we do not know how to change. Learning how to do something or how something works is important. I tried to give you all the information I wish I knew before I started my weight loss journey. It took me years to learn through trial and error, but it's what worked for me. I encourage you to do your research; there is so much more to learn. At least now you have enough knowledge to get you started, and I hope that I can at least help one person out there in some way.

Knowledge won't do you any good if you don't do anything with it. It is never too late to start. Trust me, if I was able to do it, so can you.

Good luck. You got this.

This page was intentionally left blank

This page was intentionally left blank, again...